## Table of Contents

# INTRODUCTION

Garcinia kola (bitter kola), also known as African wonder nut, belongs to the family guttiferae and grows in coastal rainforests in the South-Western and South-Eastern parts of Nigeria. Traditionally, the nuts of bitter kola are chewed as masticatory substance to stimulate the flow of saliva. The kernels of the nuts are widely traded and eaten as a stimulant. Bitter kola is also highly valued because of its medicinal benefits. The nuts are chewed for aphrodisiac effects or used to cure cough-dysentery or chest cold in herbal medicine.

In this present day, new initiatives in pharmaceutical and also livestock industries are seeking to promote the use of alternative materials that combine the effects of nutritional and medicinal properties, simultaneously. This is expected among others benefits to reduce the high cost of production in the livestock industry as a result of the reduction in dual costs of feed and drugs. Further research was made into indigenous fruits trees or plants that possesses both nutritional and medicinal properties. Bitter kola been a plant that possesses both medicinal and nutritive value and every more was emerged, and further investigations based on its current information in relation to its nutritional and medicinal properties has been aggregated.

This seeks to aggregate current information on the characteristics of bitter kola based on its history and origin as an indigenous medicinal plant in the rain forest of central and western African. Its botanical and agronomical characteristics are also discussed further; the bitter kola tree produces reddish yellowish or orange coloured fruit with each fruit containing two or four yellow seeds and a sour tasting pulp. During cultivation of bitter kola, it is either cultivated by seeds or by cutting, by the preparation of a suitable seed bed for planting and germination or by cutting from very tender branches and stems with young healthy leaves.

The nutrient and chemical composition of bitter kola as reported were also illustrated based on their various constituents. The moisture content, protein, fiber, ash and nitrogen free extracts have various amount of percentage dry matter and they are 14.60% 0.58%, 0.10%, 5.00%, 91.32% and 57.54% respectively and the vitamins as well as mineral composition also have various dry weight basis. The phytochemicals constituents of bitter kola as described are phenols (0.11 mg/100g), Alkaloids (0.36mg/100g), tannins (0.26mg/100g) and flavonoids (1.98mg/100g).

Bitter kola basically performs various other functions like medicinal uses e.g helps in weight loss, treats arthritics, anti-poison, diabetes, malaria etc.

# WHAT IS DIABETES?

Diabetes is a common disease that affects our bodies' regulation of blood sugar known as glucose. As a vital source of energy, glucose powers muscular and tissue cells, and it's a central supply of fuel for our brain. The insulin hormone - created by the pancreas - helps to draw glucose from the foods we eat and into our cells for energy.

At times, our body may not produce enough insulin to use glucose properly; the sugar then stays within the blood. By having too much blood sugar, diabetes can develop and lead to serious health complications and even death. Currently, there are no cures for diabetes; however, there are standard methods for managing diabetes and maintain health

Diabetes is a disease that occurs when your blood glucose, also called blood sugar, is too high. Blood glucose is your main source of energy and comes from the food you eat. Insulin, a hormone made by the pancreas, helps glucose from food get into your cells to be used for energy. Sometimes your body doesn't make enough—or any—insulin or doesn't use insulin well. Glucose then stays in your blood and doesn't reach your cells.

Over time, having too much glucose in your blood can cause health problems. Although diabetes has no cure, you can take steps to manage your diabetes and stay healthy.

Sometimes people call diabetes "a touch of sugar" or "borderline diabetes." These terms suggest that someone doesn't really have diabetes or has a less serious case, but every case of diabetes is serious.

## Types of Diabetes

The most common types of diabetes are type 1, type 2, and gestational diabetes.

### Type 1 diabetes

If you have type 1 diabetes, your body does not make insulin. Your immune system attacks and destroys the cells in your pancreas that make insulin. Type 1 diabetes is usually diagnosed in children and young adults, although it can appear at any age. People with type 1 diabetes need to take insulin every day to stay alive.

## *What is type 1 diabetes?*

Diabetes occurs when your blood glucose, also called blood sugar, is too high. Blood glucose is your main source of energy and comes mainly from the food you eat. Insulin, a hormone made by the pancreas, helps the glucose in your blood get into your cells to be used for energy. Another hormone, glucagon, works with insulin to control blood glucose levels.

## *Who is more likely to develop type 1 diabetes?*

Type 1 diabetes typically occurs in children and young adults, although it can appear at any age. Having a parent or sibling with the disease may increase your chance of developing type 1 diabetes. In the United States, about 5 percent of people with diabetes have type 1.[1]

Symptoms of type 1 diabetes are serious and usually happen quickly, over a few days to weeks. Symptoms can include

- increased thirst and urination
- increased hunger
- blurred vision
- fatigue
- unexplained weight loss

Sometimes the first symptoms of type 1 diabetes are signs of a life-threatening condition called diabetic ketoacidosis (DKA) . Some symptoms of DKA include

- breath that smells fruity
- dry or flushed skin
- nausea or vomiting
- stomach pain
- trouble breathing
- trouble paying attention or feeling confused

DKA is serious and dangerous. If you or your child have symptoms of DKA, contact your health care professional right away, or go to the nearest hospital emergency room.

*What causes type 1 diabetes?*

Experts think type 1 diabetes is caused by genes and factors in the environment, such as viruses, that might trigger the disease. Researchers are working to pinpoint the causes of type 1 diabetes through studies such as TrialNet .

How do health care professionals diagnose type 1 diabetes?

Health care professionals usually test people for type 1 diabetes if they have clear-cut diabetes symptoms. Health care professionals most often use the random plasma glucose (RPG) test to diagnose type 1 diabetes. This blood test measures your blood glucose level at a single point in time. Sometimes health professionals also use the A1C blood test to find out how long someone has had high blood glucose.

Even though these tests can confirm that you have diabetes, they can't identify what type you have. Treatment depends on the type of diabetes, so knowing whether you have type 1 or type 2 is important.

To find out if your diabetes is type 1, your health care professional may test your blood for certain autoantibodies. Autoantibodies are antibodies that attack your healthy tissues and cells by mistake. The presence of certain types of autoantibodies is common in type 1 but not in type 2 diabetes.

Because type 1 diabetes can run in families, your health care professional can test your family members for autoantibodies. Type 1 diabetes TrialNet, an international research network, also offers autoantibody testing to family members of people diagnosed with the disease. The presence of autoantibodies, even without diabetes symptoms, means the family member is more likely to develop type 1 diabetes. If you have a brother or sister, child, or parent with type 1 diabetes, you may want to get an autoantibody test. People age 20 or younger who have a cousin, aunt, uncle, niece, nephew, grandparent, or half-sibling with type 1 diabetes also may want to get tested.

What health problems can people with type 1 diabetes develop?

Over time, high blood glucose leads to problems such as

- heart disease
- stroke
- kidney disease
- eye problems
- dental disease
- nerve damage
- foot problems
- depression
- sleep apnea

If you have type 1 diabetes, you can help prevent or delay the health problems of diabetes by managing your blood glucose, blood pressure, and cholesterol, and following your self-care plan.

## What is type 2 diabetes?

Type 2 diabetes, the most common type of diabetes, is a disease that occurs when your blood glucose, also called blood sugar, is too high. Blood glucose is your main source of energy and comes mainly from the food you eat. Insulin, a hormone made by the pancreas, helps glucose get into your cells to be used for energy. In type 2 diabetes, your body doesn't make enough insulin or doesn't use insulin well. Too much glucose then stays in your blood, and not enough reaches your cells.

The good news is that you can take steps to prevent or delay the development of type 2 diabetes.

## Who is more likely to develop type 2 diabetes?

You can develop type 2 diabetes at any age, even during childhood. However, type 2 diabetes occurs most often in middle-aged and older people. You are more likely to develop type 2 diabetes if you are age 45 or older, have a family history of diabetes, or are overweight or obese.

Diabetes is more common in people who are African American, Hispanic/Latino, American Indian, Asian American, or Pacific Islander.

Physical inactivity and certain health problems such as high blood pressure affect your chances of developing type 2 diabetes. You are also more likely to develop type 2 diabetes if you have prediabetes or had gestational diabetes when you were pregnant. Learn more about risk factors for type 2 diabetes.

*Type 2 diabetes*

If you have type 2 diabetes, your body does not make or use insulin well. You can develop type 2 diabetes at any age, even during childhood. However, this type of diabetes occurs most often in middle-aged and older people. Type 2 is the most common type of diabetes.

*Gestational diabetes*

Gestational diabetes develops in some women when they are pregnant. Most of the time, this type of diabetes goes away after the baby is born. However, if you've had gestational diabetes, you have a greater chance of developing type 2 diabetes later in life. Sometimes diabetes diagnosed during pregnancy is actually type 2 diabetes.

*Other types of diabetes*

Less common types include monogenic diabetes, which is an inherited form of diabetes, and cystic fibrosis-related diabetes .

*How common is diabetes?*

As of 2015, 30.3 million people in the United States, or 9.4 percent of the population, had diabetes. More than 1 in 4 of them didn't know they had the disease. Diabetes affects 1 in 4 people over the age of 65. About 90-95 percent of cases in adults are type 2 diabetes.[1]

*Who is more likely to develop type 2 diabetes?*

You are more likely to develop type 2 diabetes if you are age 45 or older, have a family history of diabetes, or are overweight. Physical inactivity, race, and certain health problems such as high blood pressure also affect your chance of developing type 2 diabetes. You are also more likely to develop type 2 diabetes if you have prediabetes or had gestational diabetes when you were pregnant. Learn more about risk factors for type 2 diabetes.

*What health problems can people with diabetes develop?*

Over time, high blood glucose leads to problems such as

- heart disease
- stroke
- kidney disease
- eye problems
- dental disease
- nerve damage
- foot problems

You can take steps to lower your chances of developing these diabetes-related health

## What are the symptoms of diabetes?

- increased thirst and urination
- increased hunger
- fatigue
- blurred vision
- numbness or tingling in the feet or hands
- sores that do not heal
- unexplained weight loss

Symptoms of type 1 diabetes can start quickly, in a matter of weeks. Symptoms of type 2 diabetes often develop slowly—over the course of several years—and can be so mild that you might not even notice them. Many people with type 2 diabetes have no symptoms. Some people do not find out they have the disease until they have diabetes-related health problems, such as blurred vision or heart trouble.

## What causes type 1 diabetes?

Type 1 diabetes occurs when your immune system, the body's system for fighting infection, attacks and destroys the insulin-producing beta cells of the pancreas. Scientists think type 1 diabetes is caused by genes and environmental factors, such as viruses, that might trigger the disease. Studies such as TrialNet are working to pinpoint causes of type 1 diabetes and possible ways to prevent or slow the disease.

## What causes type 2 diabetes?

Type 2 diabetes—the most common form of diabetes—is caused by several factors, including lifestyle factors and genes.

### Overweight, obesity, and physical inactivity

You are more likely to develop type 2 diabetes if you are not physically active and are overweight or obese. Extra weight sometimes causes insulin resistance and is common in people with type 2 diabetes. The location of body fat also makes a difference. Extra belly fat is linked to insulin resistance, type 2 diabetes, and heart and blood vessel disease. To see if your weight puts you at risk for type 2 diabetes, check out these Body Mass Index (BMI) charts.

## Insulin resistance

Type 2 diabetes usually begins with insulin resistance, a condition in which muscle, liver, and fat cells do not use insulin well. As a result, your body needs more insulin to help glucose enter cells. At first, the pancreas makes more insulin to keep up with the added demand. Over time, the pancreas can't make enough insulin, and blood glucose levels rise.

## Genes and family history

As in type 1 diabetes, certain genes may make you more likely to develop type 2 diabetes. The disease tends to run in families and occurs more often in these racial/ethnic groups:

- African Americans
- Alaska Natives
- American Indians
- Asian Americans

- Hispanics/Latinos
- Native Hawaiians
- Pacific Islanders

Genes also can increase the risk of type 2 diabetes by increasing a person's tendency to become overweight or obese.

## What causes gestational diabetes?

Scientists believe gestational diabetes, a type of diabetes that develops during pregnancy, is caused by the hormonal changes of pregnancy along with genetic and lifestyle factors.

### *Insulin resistance*

Hormones produced by the placenta contribute to insulin resistance, which occurs in all women during late pregnancy. Most pregnant women can produce enough insulin to overcome insulin resistance, but some cannot. Gestational diabetes occurs when the pancreas can't make enough insulin.

As with type 2 diabetes, **extra weight** is linked to gestational diabetes. Women who are overweight or obese may already have insulin resistance when they become pregnant. Gaining too much weight during pregnancy may also be a factor.

## *Genes and family history*

Having a family history of diabetes makes it more likely that a woman will develop gestational diabetes, which suggests that genes play a role. Genes may also explain why the disorder occurs more often in African Americans, American Indians, Asians, and Hispanics/Latinas.

## What else can cause diabetes?

Genetic mutations , other diseases, damage to the pancreas, and certain medicines may also cause diabetes.

## *Genetic mutations*

- Monogenic diabetes is caused by mutations, or changes, in a single gene. These changes are usually passed through families, but sometimes the gene mutation happens on its own. Most of these gene mutations cause diabetes by making the pancreas less able to make insulin. The most common types of monogenic diabetes are neonatal diabetes and maturity-onset diabetes of the young (MODY). Neonatal diabetes occurs in the first 6 months of life. Doctors usually diagnose MODY during adolescence or early adulthood, but sometimes the disease is not diagnosed until later in life.

Cystic fibrosis produces thick mucus that causes scarring in the pancreas. This scarring can prevent the pancreas from making enough insulin.

Hemochromatosis causes the body to store too much iron. If the disease is not treated, iron can build up in and damage the pancreas and other organs.

*Hormonal diseases*

Some hormonal diseases cause the body to produce too much of certain hormones, which sometimes cause insulin resistance and diabetes.

- Cushing's syndrome occurs when the body produces too much cortisol—often called the "stress hormone."
- Acromegaly occurs when the body produces too much growth hormone.
- Hyperthyroidism occurs when the thyroid gland produces too much thyroid hormone.

Damage to or removal of the pancreas

Pancreatitis, pancreatic cancer, and trauma can all harm the beta cells or make them less able to produce insulin, resulting in diabetes. If the damaged pancreas is removed, diabetes will occur due to the loss of the beta cells.

*Medicines*

Sometimes certain medicines can harm beta cells or disrupt the way insulin works. These include

- niacin, a type of vitamin B3
- certain types of diuretics, also called water pills
- anti-seizure drugs

- psychiatric drugs

- drugs to treat human immunodeficiency virus (HIV )

- pentamidine, a drug used to treat a type of pneumonia

- glucocorticoids—medicines used to treat inflammatory illnesses such as rheumatoid arthritis , asthma , lupus , and ulcerative colitis

- anti-rejection medicines, used to help stop the body from rejecting a transplanted organ

Statins, which are medicines to reduce LDL ("bad") cholesterol levels, can slightly increase the chance that you'll develop diabetes. However, statins help protect you from heart disease and stroke. For this reason, the strong benefits of taking statins outweigh the small chance that you could develop diabetes.

## Risk Factors for Type 2 Diabetes

Your chances of developing type 2 diabetes depend on a combination of risk factors such as your genes and lifestyle. Although you can't change risk factors such as family history, age, or ethnicity, you can change lifestyle risk factors around eating, physical activity, and weight. These lifestyle changes can affect your chances of developing type 2 diabetes.

Read about risk factors for type 2 diabetes below and see which ones apply to you. Taking action on the factors you can change can help you delay or prevent type 2 diabetes.

You are more likely to develop type 2 diabetes if you

- are overweight or obese
- are age 45 or older
- have a family history of diabetes
- are African American, Alaska Native, American Indian, Asian American, Hispanic/Latino, Native Hawaiian, or Pacific Islander
- have high blood pressure
- have a low level of HDL ("good") cholesterol, or a high level of triglycerides

- have a history of gestational diabetes or gave birth to a baby weighing 9 pounds or more
- are not physically active
- have a history of heart disease or stroke
- have depression
- have polycystic ovary syndrome , also called PCOS
- have acanthosis nigricans—dark, thick, and velvety skin around your neck or armpits

You can also take the Diabetes Risk Test to learn about your risk for type 2 diabetes.

To see if your weight puts you at risk for type 2 diabetes, find your height in the Body Mass Index (BMI) charts below. If your weight is equal to or more than the weight listed, you have a greater chance of developing the disease.

If you are not Asian American or Pacific Islander

If you are Asian American

If you are Pacific Islander

| At-risk BMI ≥ 25 | | At-risk BMI ≥ 23 | | At-risk BMI ≥ 26 | |
| --- | --- | --- | --- | --- | --- |
| Height | Weight | Height | Weight | Height | Weight |
| 4'10" | 119 | 4'10" | 110 | 4'10" | 124 |
| 4'11" | 124 | 4'11" | 114 | 4'11" | 128 |
| 5'0" | 128 | 5'0" | 118 | 5'0" | 133 |
| 5'1" | 132 | 5'1" | 122 | 5'1" | 137 |
| 5'2" | 136 | 5'2" | 126 | 5'2" | 142 |
| 5'3" | 141 | 5'3" | 130 | 5'3" | 146 |
| 5'4" | 145 | 5'4" | 134 | 5'4" | 151 |
| 5'5" | 150 | 5'5" | 138 | 5'5" | 156 |
| 5'6" | 155 | 5'6" | 142 | 5'6" | 161 |
| 5'7" | 159 | 5'7" | 146 | 5'7" | 166 |
| 5'8" | 164 | 5'8" | 151 | 5'8" | 171 |

| If you are not Asian American or Pacific Islander | | If you are Asian American | | If you are Pacific Islander | |
| --- | --- | --- | --- | --- | --- |
| At-risk BMI ≥ 25 | | At-risk BMI ≥ 23 | | At-risk BMI ≥ 26 | |
| Height | Weight | Height | Weight | Height | Weight |
| 5'9" | 169 | 5'9" | 155 | 5'9" | 176 |
| 5'10" | 174 | 5'10" | 160 | 5'10" | 181 |
| 5'11" | 179 | 5'11" | 165 | 5'11" | 186 |
| 6'0" | 184 | 6'0" | 169 | 6'0" | 191 |
| 6'1" | 189 | 6'1" | 174 | 6'1" | 197 |
| 6'2" | 194 | 6'2" | 179 | 6'2" | 202 |
| 6'3" | 200 | 6'3" | 184 | 6'3" | 208 |
| 6'4" | 205 | 6'4" | 189 | 6'4" | 213 |

You can take steps to help prevent or delay type 2 diabetes by losing weight if you are overweight, eating fewer calories, and being more physically active. Talk with your health care professional about any of the health conditions listed above that may require medical treatment. Managing these health problems may help reduce your chances of developing type 2 diabetes. Also, ask your health care professional about any medicines you take that might increase your risk.

What tests are used to diagnose diabetes and prediabetes?

Health care professionals most often use the fasting plasma glucose (FPG) test or the A1C test to diagnose diabetes. In some cases, they may use a random plasma glucose (RPG) test.

*Fasting plasma glucose (FPG) test*

The FPG blood test measures your blood glucose level at a single point in time. For the most reliable results, it is best to have this test in the morning, after you fast for at least 8 hours. Fasting means having nothing to eat or drink except sips of water.



*A1C test*

The A1C test is a blood test that provides your average levels of blood glucose over the past 3 months. Other names for the A1C test are hemoglobin A1C, HbA1C, glycated hemoglobin, and glycosylated hemoglobin test. You can eat and drink before this test. When it comes to using the A1C to diagnose diabetes, your doctor will consider factors such as your age and whether you have anemia or another problem with your blood.[1] The A1C test is not accurate in people with anemia.

If you're of African, Mediterranean, or Southeast Asian descent, your A1C test results may be falsely high or low. Your health care professional may need to order a different type of A1C test.

Your health care professional will report your A1C test result as a percentage, such as an A1C of 7 percent. The higher the percentage, the higher your average blood glucose levels.

People with diabetes also use information from the A1C test to help manage their diabetes.

*Random plasma glucose (RPG) test*

Sometimes health care professionals use the RPG test to diagnose diabetes when diabetes symptoms are present and they do not want to wait until you have fasted. You do not need to fast overnight for the RPG test. You may have this blood test at any time.

What tests are used to diagnose gestational diabetes?

Pregnant women may have the glucose challenge test, the oral glucose tolerance test, or both. These tests show how well your body handles glucose.

*Glucose challenge test*

If you are pregnant and a health care professional is checking you for gestational diabetes, you may first receive the glucose challenge test. Another name for this test is the glucose screening test. In this test, a health care professional will draw your blood 1 hour after you drink a sweet liquid containing glucose. You do not need to fast for this test. If your blood glucose is too high—135 to 140 or more—you may need to return for an oral glucose tolerance test while fasting.

*Oral glucose tolerance test (OGTT)*

The OGTT measures blood glucose after you fast for at least 8 hours. First, a health care professional will draw your blood. Then you will drink the liquid containing glucose. For diagnosing gestational diabetes, you will need your blood drawn every hour for 2 to 3 hours.

High blood glucose levels at any two or more blood test times during the OGTT—fasting, 1 hour, 2 hours, or 3 hours—mean you have gestational diabetes. Your health care team will explain what your OGTT results mean.

Health care professionals also can use the OGTT to diagnose type 2 diabetes and prediabetes in people who are not pregnant. The OGTT helps health care professionals detect type 2 diabetes and prediabetes better than the FPG test. However, the OGTT is a more expensive test and is not as easy to give. To diagnose type 2 diabetes and prediabetes, a health care professional will need to draw your blood 1 hour after you drink the liquid containing glucose and again after 2 hours.

What test numbers tell me if I have diabetes or prediabetes?

Each test to detect diabetes and prediabetes uses a different measurement. Usually, the same test method needs to be repeated on a second day to diagnose diabetes. Your doctor may also use a second test method to confirm that you have diabetes.

gestational diabetes, health care professionals give more glucose to drink and use different numbers as cutoffs.

Source: Adapted from American Diabetes Association. Classification and diagnosis of diabetes. Diabetes Care. 2016;39(1):S14–S20, tables 2.1, 2.3.

Which tests help my health care professional know what kind of diabetes I have?

Even though the tests described here can confirm that you have diabetes, they can't identify what type you have. Sometimes health care professionals are unsure if diabetes is type 1 or type 2. A rare type of diabetes that can occur in babies, called monogenic diabetes, can also be mistaken for type 1 diabetes. Treatment depends on the type of diabetes, so knowing which type you have is important.

To find out if your diabetes is type 1, your health care professional may look for certain autoantibodies. Autoantibodies are antibodies that mistakenly attack your healthy tissues and cells. The presence of one or more of several types of autoantibodies specific to diabetes is common in type 1 diabetes, but not in type 2 or monogenic diabetes. A health care professional will have to draw your blood for this test.

If you had diabetes while you were pregnant, you should get tested no later than 12 weeks after your baby is born to see if you have type 2 diabetes.

## Symptoms of Diabetes

Diabetes symptoms are caused by rising blood sugar.

### General symptoms

The general symptoms of diabetes include:

- increased hunger
- increased thirst
- weight loss
- frequent urination
- blurry vision
- extreme fatigue
- sores that don't heal

## Symptoms in men

In addition to the general symptoms of diabetes, men with diabetes may have a decreased sex drive, erectile dysfunction (ED), and poor muscle strength.

**Symptoms in women**

Women with diabetes can also have symptoms such as urinary tract infections, yeast infections, and dry, itchy skin.

*Type 1 diabetes*

Symptoms of type 1 diabetes can include:

- extreme hunger
- increased thirst
- unintentional weight loss
- frequent urination
- blurry vision
- tiredness

It may also result in mood changes.

*Type 2 diabetes*

Symptoms of type 2 diabetes can include:

- increased hunger
- increased thirst

- increased urination

- blurry vision

- tiredness

- sores that are slow to heal

It may also cause recurring infections. This is because elevated glucose levels make it harder for the body to heal.

## Gestational diabetes

Most women with gestational diabetes don't have any symptoms. The condition is often detected during a routine blood sugar test or oral glucose tolerance test that is usually performed between the 24th and 28th weeks of gestation.

In rare cases, a woman with gestational diabetes will also experience increased thirst or urination.

## Causes of Diabetes

Different causes are associated with each type of diabetes.

*Type 1 diabetes*

Doctors don't know exactly what causes type 1 diabetes. For some reason, the immune system mistakenly attacks and destroys insulin-producing beta cells in the pancreas.

Genes may play a role in some people. It's also possible that a virus sets off the immune system attack.

*Type 2 diabetes*

Type 2 diabetes stems from a combination of genetics and lifestyle factors. Being overweight or obese increases your risk too. Carrying extra weight, especially in your belly, makes your cells more resistant to the effects of insulin on your blood sugar.

This condition runs in families. Family members share genes that make them more likely to get type 2 diabetes and to be overweight.

*Gestational diabetes*

Gestational diabetes is the result of hormonal changes during pregnancy. The placenta produces hormones that make a pregnant woman's cells less sensitive to the effects of insulin. This can cause high blood sugar during pregnancy.

Women who are overweight when they get pregnant or who gain too much weight during their pregnancy are more likely to get gestational diabetes.

The bottom line

Both genes and environmental factors play a role in triggering diabetes.

## Diabetes Diagnosis

Anyone who has symptoms of diabetes or is at risk for the disease should be tested. Women are routinely tested for gestational diabetes during their second or third trimesters of pregnancy.

Doctors use these blood tests to diagnose prediabetes and diabetes:

- The fasting plasma glucose (FPG) test measures your blood sugar after you've fasted for 8 hours.
- The A1C test provides a snapshot of your blood sugar levels over the previous 3 months.

To diagnose gestational diabetes, your doctor will test your blood sugar levels between the 24th and 28th weeks of your pregnancy.

- During the glucose challenge test, your blood sugar is checked an hour after you drink a sugary liquid.
- During the 3 hour glucose tolerance test, your blood sugar is checked after you fast overnight and then drink a sugary liquid.

The earlier you get diagnosed with diabetes, the sooner you can start treatment. Find out whether you should get tested, and get more information on tests your doctor might perform.

# GARCINIA KOLA/BITTER KOLA

Garcinia Kola popularly called Bitter Kola is a bitter traditional fruit common in the West Africa and it is generally considered medicinal with no effects.

Garcinia Kola belongs to the species of a tropical flowering plant that produces brown nut like seeds. Traditionally, the fruit, seeds, nuts and the bark of the bitter kola plant have been used for centuries for herbal medicine to treat several ailments.

This bitter kola, which is believed to contain a high source of vitamins and minerals such as Vitamins A, C, E, B1, B2, B3, fiber, calcium, potassium, and iron, also carry other antioxidants and the usage is not limited to traditional activities alone.

Bitter Kola was eaten mostly by the elderly people because of their belief that it could prolong life. Imperatively, researchers in modern science have revealed that bitter kola contains chemical compounds that will help the breakdown of glycogen in the liver and has other medicinal uses which account for its longevity properties in man.

History has it that Garcinia kola is a specie of flowering plant in the Clusiaceae or Guttiferae family. It is found in Benin, Cameroon, Republic of Congo, Ivory Coast, Ghana, Gabon, Senegal, Liberia, Sierra Leone and Nigeria. This natural habitat is subtropical or tropical moist lowland forests.

It has been used for centuries in folk medicine to treat ailments from coughs to fever. According to a report from the Center For International Forestry Research, Garcinia kola trade is still important to the indigenous communities and villages in Nigeria.

## Health Benefits of Bitter Kola

It is possible to use bitter kola to improve several medical conditions for a short period. This might work for depressions, fatigue problems, atonic diarrhea, migraine, and other disease conditions.

Bitter Kola tree have been widely used both in medicine and in cosmetology due to their stimulating, astringent, draining, decongestant, antioxidant, anti-inflammatory, vaso-protective, lipolytic and a number of other properties. Health benefits of bitter kola make it a fair alternative for a list of pills and medicines.

## Bitter kola serve as remedy for osteoarthritis

Osteoarthritis is the most common form of arthritis, affecting millions of people worldwide. It occurs when the protective cartilage that cushions the ends of your bones wears down over time.

Although osteoarthritis can damage any joint, the disorder most commonly affects joints in your hands, knees, hips and spine.

## Bitter kola helps to combat sexually transmitted diseases (STDs)

The term sexually transmitted disease (STD) is used to refer to a condition passed from one person to another through sexual contact. You can contract an STD by having unprotected vaginal, anal, or oral sex with someone who has the STD.

An STD may also be called a sexually transmitted infection (STI) or venereal disease (VD).

That doesn't mean sex is the only way STDs are transmitted. Depending on the specific STD, infections may also be transmitted through sharing needles and breastfeeding.

## Bitter kola helps to improves immune system

Bitter kola provide the immune system with all the needed supports in order to protect one from attacks of harmful toxins and effective immune response against strange particles.

This high amount of antioxidants found in bitter kola does not only help fight bacteria and other illnesses, it also helps the body to increase its immunity levels.

And when the immunity level of the body is increased, it becomes strong enough to fight against any foreign contaminant.

## Bitter kola helps cure impotence

With bitter kola impotent is an history because studies have shown that when it comes to the improvement of sexual performance, especially among men, bitter kola is king among all other suggested herbs.

Bitter Kola does not only increase sex drive, it also improves the sexual performance of men who consume it. Research indicate that for the seed to be effective, it is advisable for the seed to be chewed some minutes before the intercourse.

It has also been confirmed that bitter kola helps to increase sperm counts and promote male fertility, which can be useful for those of you out there looking into adding a little one to your family.

Not only that, but bitter kola can actually help to boost libido in men as well. It's a potent aphrodisiac and studies have shown it can actually temporarily boost testosterone levels.

## Bitter kola aids proper functioning of the lungs

The fibers and lung tissues are not only strengthened when bitter kola is consumed regularly in a considerate amount, it also stabilises any other counter effect.

In addition, it helps in the maintenance of good respiratory tract as well as treating chest cold. It has a favourably high antioxidant content for a healthy body.

Bitter kola's benefit to lung properties are attributed to its high antioxidant content. So, if you are a smoker or even a passive smoker, definitely bitter kola is the cure.

## Bitter kola fights Glaucoma (eye pressure)

Glaucoma, known as eye pressure is a condition of increased pressure within the eyeball, causing a gradual loss of sight. Glaucoma could result in permanent blindness if left untreated.

However, bitter kola has been found to be an amazing remedy for the eye. "when bitter kola is eaten, at least twice a day, it could successfully reduce the eye pressure".

## Bitter kola helps reduce constipation

Kola nut functions as a dietary fibre in food as it helps in the prevention and treatments of health conditions that relate to the digestive system which includes but is not limited to bloating, constipation and other conditions that disrupt the bowel movement.

## Bitter kola enhances cancer treatment

Bitter kola have been found effective in stopping growing of tumours and cancerous disease in human body. Researches show that the presence of a chemical compound known as phytoestrogens in bitter kola is used for cancer treatment and reduce the growth of tumour cells.

Similarly, there is a non-steroidal plant compound contained in kola nut extracts which have the ability to terminate the growth and development of prostate cancer cells in the body.

## Bitter kola increases mental alertness

The caffeine content in bitter kola makes it a good stimulant or psycho-stimulants for the central nervous system; as it helps to improve awareness, mood and elevated mood.

These nuts, specifically bitter kola are regarded as cognitive boosters.

## Bitter kola helps promotes diuresis

Kola nuts and bitter kola contain bitter chemicals such as caffeine and theobromine which serve as natural diuretics. This implies that the bitter content in these nuts helps to increase water and salt expelled from human body; and some minor sicknesses in the body are flushed out through urine in the process which makes them beneficial to human health.

Bitter kola isn't just useful for treating malaria. It can also be effective for individuals who have type 2 diabetes as a means of keeping their blood glucose levels stable.

# BITTER KOLA FOR DIABETES

Bitter kola and diabetes: Does it help? Speaking about its role in curing diabetes, it can be said that effect of bitter kola on diabetes can be rather impressive. As for bitter kola for diabetes, it has been proven that bitter kola can regulate the level of sugar in blood and can cope with an elevated level of sugar – reducing and normalizing it. Read more: https://www.legit.ng/1083822-bitter-kola-diabetes-does.html

According to legit.ng, bitter kola has a unique chemical composition which could explain its medicinal benefits:

The Kola nut includes caffeine, theophylline, theobromine, sugar, water, starch, cellulose, and phenolic compounds:

• phlobaphene;

• tannic acid;

• catechins and epicatechin.

It also increases the metabolism and extracts derived from the nut can increase the speed of metabolic processes as well as speeding up heart rate. However, this effect is achieved at low concentrations and low doses. In large doses it increases the risk of heart failure so one has to be careful with their dosage.

The effect of bitter kola on diabetes are quite astounding. It has been proven that bitter kola can regulate blood sugar levels in blood by reducing and normalising it, with prolonged use.

Those who suffer from the negative effects of elevated blood sugar can find some relief with bitter kola. Kola nut efficiently regulates the amount of sugar in your blood, relieving you from the discomfort of diabetes.

However, it's worth noting that in serious cases of diabetes it's recommended to combine the use of bitter kola with the use of medicine prescribed by the doctor. Because it's difficult to understand dosage and effect when it comes to native medicine, make sure you consult your doctor before using natural solutions.

## Doseage

Taking it an hour before or after meals may help to increase the absorption of the key ingredients. Food does not affect the metabolism of Garcinia kola and may buffer effects of mild indigestion.

## Side effects of bitter kola

Consumption of bitter kola nuts is completely safe. I personally haven't experienced any sort of side effects or anything like that with eating bitter kola.

# CONCLUSION

Studies have found that the seeds from the plant are capable of reducing elevated blood glucose levels. This makes it ideal for both treatment of type 2 diabetes as well as for any complications that can arise from the condition.

Bitter kola isn't just useful for treating malaria. It can also be effective for individuals who have type 2 diabetes as a means of keeping their blood glucose levels stable.